The Step-by-Step Instant Pot Cookbook

Simple and Delicious Recipes for Your Instant Pot

Felicity Brown

Sommario

Introduction 7

Lunch 9

  California Sandwich 9

  Miso Soup 11

  Chicken Burrito 13

  Lettuce and Tuna Salad 16

  Carrots Casserole 18

  Home Lunch Baguette 20

  Italian Tart 23

  Warm Lunch Tortillas 25

  Quick Pie 28

  Filo Snail 31

  Puff Rolls 33

  Garlic Spaghetti 35

  Salmon Pie 37

  Onion French Soup 39

  Gnocchi 41

  Mozzarella Pie 44

  Herbed Chicken Wings 46

  Halloumi Salad with Beef Tenderloins 48

  Basil Pho 50

  Butter Asparagus Pie 52

  Enoki Mushroom Soup 54

  Mushroom Cream Soup 57

  Cauliflower Cottage Slice 59

Turkey Apple Salad 61

Ground Meat Chop 64

Provolone Pepper Soup 66

Jalapeno Garlic Soup 68

Eggplant Lasagna with Mozzarella 71

Keto Cauliflower Soup 73

Chili Egg Soup 75

Beef Soup 77

Hot Spinach Chowder 79

Butternut Ginger Soup 81

Tortilla Soup 84

Steak Zucchini Soup 86

Chili Meat 88

Garlic Taco Soup 90

Chicken Chipotle Soup 92

Creamy Cheddar Soup 94

Sausage Soup 97

Bone Broth Soup 99

Celery Chicken Soup 101

Cream & Vegetable Stew 103

Broccoli Lunch Bowl 105

Cabbage Salad 107

Cucumber and Lobster Salad 110

Italian Salad 112

Egg Salad and Cheddar with Dill 114

Cream Cheese Salad 116

Chicken Paprika..118
Conclusion...120

Introduction

This total and valuable overview to instantaneous pot cooking with over 1000 dishes for morning meal, supper, supper, and also even treats! This is just one of the most thorough split second pot cookbooks ever published thanks to its variety as well as accurate instructions.

Ingenious dishes and also standards, contemporary take on household's most liked meals-- all this is yummy, easy and also of course as healthy as it can be. Adjustment the method you prepare with these ingenious instant pot instructions. Need a brand-new dinner or a treat? Here you are! Best instantaneous pot meals collaborated in a couple of straightforward steps, also a newbie can do it! The instantaneous pot defines the way you prepare every day. This immediate pot recipe book helps you make the absolute most out of your once a week food selection. The only instant pot publication you will certainly ever before require with the supreme collection of recipes will certainly help you in the direction of a less complex and healthier kitchen area experience. If you want to save time cooking meals more successfully, if you wish to offer your household food that can please even the pickiest eater, you are in the right place! Master your immediate pot as well as make your food preparation needs fit into your busy way of life.

Lunch

California Sandwich

Prep time: 10 minutes

Cooking time: 4 minutes

Servings: 6

Ingredients:

- 5 ounces keto naan bread
- 1 teaspoon sesame seeds
- 1 tablespoon mustard
- 2 tablespoons lemon juice
- 3 tablespoons garlic sauce
- 5 ounces cheddar cheese
- ¼ cup sunflower sprouts
- 1 teaspoon onion powder
- 1 avocado, pitted
- 8 ounces smoked chicken
- 1 teaspoon butter

Directions:

1. Combine the mustard, lemon juice, garlic sauce, and onion powder together.

2. Stir the mixture well. Spread all the keto naan bread slices with the mustard sauce.

3. Slice cheddar cheese. Slice the avocado.

4. Chop the smoked chicken. Place the sliced cheese, avocado, and chopped smoked chicken into 3 bread slices.

5. Sprinkle it with the sesame seeds. Cover the mixture with the naan bread slices to make the sandwiches.

6. Add the butter in the pressure cooker. Transfer the sandwiches in the pressure cooker and set the mode to "Sauté."

7. Cook the sandwiches for 2 minutes on each side.

8. Transfer the cooked dish in the serving plates. Cut them in half and serve.

Nutrition: calories 264, fat 17.2, fiber 2.8, carbs 8.7, protein 18.8

Miso Soup

Prep time: 8 minutes

Cooking time: 10 minutes

Servings: 6

Ingredients:

- 1 tablespoon miso paste
- 1 teaspoon turmeric
- ½ tablespoon ground ginger
- 1 teaspoon cilantro
- 5 cups chicken stock
- 5 ounces celery stalk
- 1 teaspoon salt
- 1 tablespoon sesame seeds
- 1 teaspoon lemon zest
- ½ cup of soy sauce
- 1 white onion

Directions:

1. Combine the turmeric, ground ginger, cilantro, salt, lemon zest, and chicken stock together in the pressure cooker.

2. Peel the onion. Chop the celery stalk and white onion.

3. Add the vegetables in the pressure cooker.

4. Blend the mixture and close the lid. Set the pressure cooker mode to "Pressure," and cook for 8 minutes.

5. Add the miso paste and soy sauce.

6. Stir the mixture well until the miso paste dissolves. Cook for 2 minutes.

7. Ladle the soup into serving bowls.

Nutrition: calories 155, fat 7.3, fiber 1, carbs 14.66, protein 7

Chicken Burrito

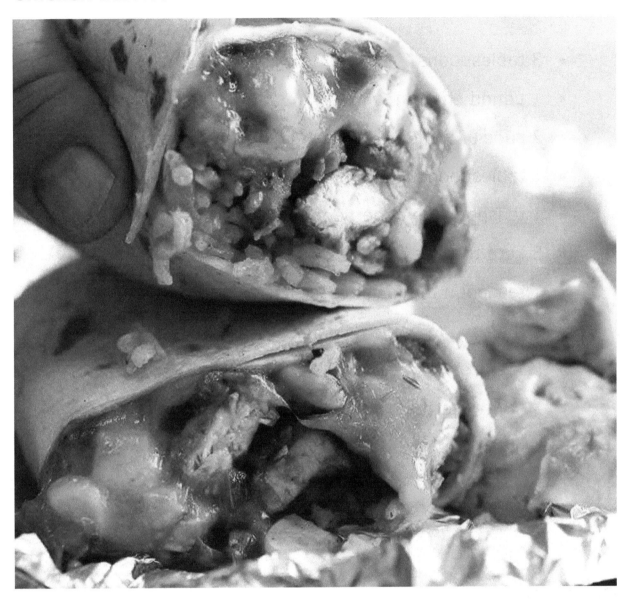

Prep time: 10 minutes

Cooking time: 35 minutes

Servings: 5

Ingredients:

- 3 tablespoons chipotle paste

- 1 pound chicken

- 2 cups of water

- 1 tablespoon tomato paste

- 1 teaspoon cayenne pepper

- 5 keto tortillas

- 1 teaspoon mayo sauce

- 1 tablespoon garlic powder

- ⅓ cup fresh parsley

- 3 ounces lettuce

- ¼ cup of salsa

Directions:

1. Chop the chicken roughly and place it in the pressure cooker. Add cayenne pepper, garlic powder, and chili pepper.

2. Pour water and close the lid. Set the pressure cooker mode to "Sear/Sauté," and cook the meat for 30 minutes.

3. Meanwhile, tear the lettuce into a mixing bowl.

4. Add salsa and mayo sauce. Blend the mixture well. Spread the keto tortillas with the salsa and chipotle paste.

5. Chop the parsley, and separate it evenly between all tortillas. Add tomato paste and lettuce mixture.

6. When the chicken is cooked, shred it well and transfer the meat in the tortillas. Wrap the tortillas to make the burritos.

7. Transfer the burritos in the pressure cooker and cook the dish on the "Sauté" mode for 5 minutes.

8. When the cooking time ends, remove the dish from the pressure cooker. Serve it immediately.

Nutrition: calories 244, fat 7.6, fiber 2.5, carbs 10.4, protein 32.6

Lettuce and Tuna Salad

Prep time: 15 minutes

Cooking time: 20 minutes

Servings: 6

Ingredients:

- 1 pound fresh tuna
- 2 red onions
- 2 bell peppers
- 1 cup lettuce
- ⅓ cup pecans
- 2 tablespoons lemon juice
- 1 teaspoon olive oil
- 2 tablespoons butter
- ½ teaspoon rosemary
- ¼ cup cream
- 5 ounces tomatoes
- 1 teaspoon salt
- ½ cup of water

Directions:

1. Sprinkle the tuna with the rosemary and salt and stir it gently.

2. Tadd the butter in the pressure cooker and add the tuna.

3. Add water and close the lid. Set the pressure cooker mode to "Pressure," and cook the fish for 20 minutes.

4. Meanwhile, peel the onions and slice them.

5. Chop the lettuce and bell peppers.

6. Chop the tomatoes and crush the pecans.

7. Place the lemon juice, olive oil, and cream in the mixing bowl and stir the mixture well. Place all the vegetables in the mixing bowl and stir the mixture gently.

8. When the tuna is cooked, remove it from the pressure cooker and shred it.

9. Add the shredded tuna in the vegetable mixture.

10. Mix up the salad using two spoons.

11. Transfer the salad in the serving bowl and sprinkle it with the cream sauce and serve it.

Nutrition: calories 190, fat 11.3, fiber 2, carbs 7.29, protein 17

Carrots Casserole

Prep time: 10 minutes

Cooking time: 40 minutes

Servings: 6

Ingredients:

- 1 pound cabbage
- 2 carrots
- 1 onion
- ½ cup tomato juice
- 5 eggs
- 1 teaspoon salt
- 1 teaspoon paprika
- ½ tablespoon coconut flour
- 1 teaspoon cilantro
- 1 tablespoon butter
- ½ cup pork rinds

Directions:

1. Chop the cabbage and sprinkle it with the salt.

2. Stir the mixture and leave it until the cabbage gives off liquid. Combine the tomato juice with the cilantro.

3. Add the butter in the pressure cooker and melt it.

4. Add the chopped cabbage and sauté it for 10 minutes, stirring frequently. Beat the eggs in the mixing bowl and whisk well.

5. Add flour and stir it until you get a smooth mixture. Add the tomato mixture in the pressure cooker and stir it well.

6. Add egg mixture and pork rinds.

7. Sprinkle the dish with the paprika.

8. Peel the onion and carrots and chop them.

9. Add the chopped ingredients in the pressure cooker and stir the mixture. Close the lid, and set the manual mode for 35 minutes.

10. When the dish is cooked, let it rest briefly and serve.

Nutrition: calories 178, fat 10, fiber 3.2, carbs 9.8, protein 13.8

Home Lunch Baguette

Prep time: 15 minutes

Cooking time: 30 minutes

Servings: 6

Ingredients:

- 2 cups almond flour
- ⅓ cup whey
- 1 teaspoon baking powder
- 1 tablespoon Erythritol
- 1 teaspoon salt
- 5 ounces Parmesan cheese
- 8 ounces Mozzarella cheese
- 1 teaspoon parsley
- 1 teaspoon cilantro
- 1 teaspoon oregano
- 1 tablespoon rosemary
- 2 eggs
- 1 tablespoon butter

- 1 cup fresh spinach

Directions:

1. Combine the whey with the baking powder and stir the mixture well.

2. Add Erythritol, salt, and cilantro and stir the mixture. Add the almond flour and knead the smooth dough.

3. Chop the parsley and combine it with the oregano. Add rosemary, eggs, and butter.

4. Chop the spinach and add it to the parsley mixture.

5. Chop the Mozzarella cheese and grate the Parmesan cheese. Combine the cheese with the green mixture and stir.

6. Fill the dough with spinach mixture and make the form of the baguette. Transfer the dish to the pressure cooker and leave it for 10 minutes.

7. Close the lid, and set the pressure cooker mode to "Pressure." Cook for 30 minutes. Turn it into another side after 15 minutes of cooking.

8. When the baguette is cooked, let it rest briefly and then remove it from the pressure cooker. Slice it and serve warm.

Nutrition: calories 285, fat 20, fiber 1.5, carbs 5.6, protein 23.6

Italian Tart

Prep time: 10 minutes

Cooking time: 25 minutes

Servings: 10

Ingredients:

- 9 ounces sundried tomatoes
- 1 teaspoon salt
- 7 ounces soda dough (keto dough)
- 1 egg yolk
- ¼ cup almond milk
- 2 tablespoons butter
- 2 white onions
- ½ cup pork rinds
- 1 teaspoon nutmeg

Directions:

1. Roll out the soda dough using a rolling pin, and transfer it to the pressure cooker.

2. Put the tomatoes in the rolled dough.

3. Peel the onions and slice them. Add the sliced onion to the tart. Sprinkle the tart with the salt.

4. Add almond milk, butter, and nutmeg. Add the pork rinds. Whisk the egg yolk and sprinkle the tart with the mixture.

5. Close the pressure cooker lid and cook for 25 minutes.

6. When the cooking time ends, release the remaining pressure and remove the tart from the pressure cooker carefully. Cut it into pieces and serve.

Nutrition: calories 218, fat 7.9, fiber 6.4, carbs 21.2, protein 19.4

Warm Lunch Tortillas

Prep time: 15 minutes

Cooking time: 10 minutes

Servings: 6

Ingredients:

- 4 eggs
- 1 teaspoon salt
- ½ teaspoon ground black pepper
- 1 tablespoon olive oil
- 6 keto tortillas
- 4 tablespoons salsa
- 1 teaspoon cilantro
- ½ teaspoon paprika
- 7 ounces beetroot
- 1 teaspoon lemon zest
- 1 medium carrot
- 1 red onion
- 1 tablespoon lemon juice

- 1 cup lettuce

Directions:

1. Beat the eggs in the mixing bowl and whisk them well.

2. Add ground black pepper, salt, cilantro, and paprika. Stir the mixture well.

3. Spray the pressure cooker inside and transfer the egg mixture. Set the pressure cooker mode to "Sauté" and ladle the egg mixture to make the crepe.

4. Cook it on each side for 1 minute. Continue this step with five additional crepes. Chill the crepes.

5. Spread the keto tortillas with the salsa. Sprinkle them with the lemon juice and add lettuce. Add the egg crepes. Cut the carrot into the strips.

6. Chop the beetroot and slice the onion.

7. Add the vegetables into the tortillas.

8. Add lemon zest and make the wraps. Transfer the wraps into the pressure cooker and cook them at the manual mode for 3 minutes.

9. Remove the dish from the pressure cooker and serve hot.

Nutrition: calories 144, fat 8.1, fiber 3, carbs 10.2, protein 8.8

Quick Pie

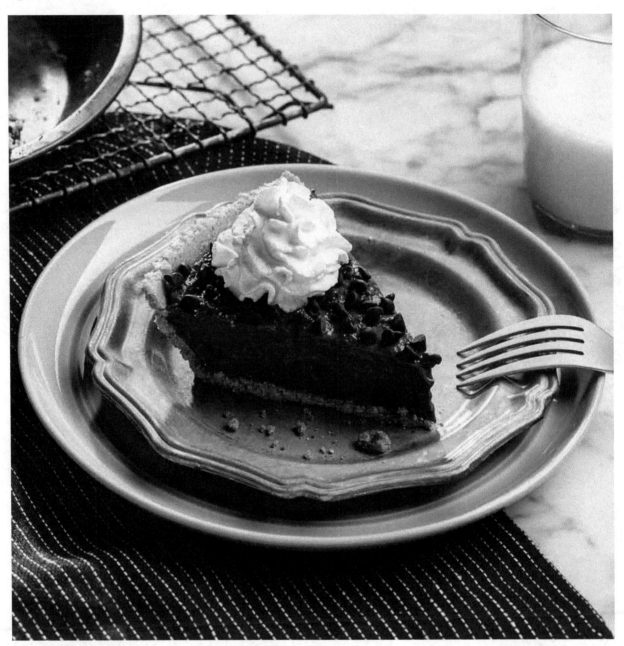

Prep time: 15 minutes

Cooking time: 25 minutes

Servings: 8

Ingredients:

- 2 cups almond flour
- 7 ounces butter
- 1 teaspoon salt
- 1 egg
- ¼ cup almond milk
- 1 pound sausage
- 1 teaspoon tomato paste
- 5 ounces Parmesan cheese
- 1 teaspoon cilantro
- 1 teaspoon oregano
- 3 tablespoons sour cream
- 1 teaspoon turmeric
- 1 carrot

Directions:

1. Combine the butter with the almond flour. Add salt, almond milk, and egg.

2. Knead the dough. Chop the sausages and combine them with the tomato paste.

3. Add the cilantro, oregano, and sour cream. Sprinkle the sausage mixture with the turmeric.

4. Peel the carrot and slice it. Roll the dough into the round form and transfer it into the pressure cooker.

5. Put the sausage mixture in the middle of the dough and flatten it well. Add the sliced carrot and milk.

6. Close the lid, and set the pressure cooker mode to "Pressure." Follow the directions of the pressure cooker. Cook for 25 minutes.

7. Check if the dish is cooked using a wooden spoon and remove it from the pressure cooker. Slice it and serve.

Nutrition: calories 615, fat 56.4, fiber 3.3, carbs 7.6, protein 23

Filo Snail

Prep time: 15 minutes

Cooking time: 30 minutes

Servings: 6

Ingredients:

- 5 sheets filo pastry
- 1 tablespoon sesame seeds
- 1 tablespoon olive oil
- 1 teaspoon butter
- 1 cup spinach
- 1 teaspoon oregano
- ½ teaspoon nutmeg
- 1 teaspoon cilantro
- 1 cup cottage cheese
- 1 teaspoon garlic powder
- 1 egg yolk

Directions:

1. Sprinkle the filo pastry sheets with the olive oil.

2. Chop the spinach and combine it with the oregano, nutmeg, cilantro, cottage cheese, and garlic powder. Stir the mixture well.

3. Place the spinach mixture into the filo pastry sheets and roll them into the shape of the snail. Whisk the egg yolk and sprinkle the "snail" with it.

4. Add sesame seeds and transfer the dish to the pressure cooker.

5. Close the lid, and set the pressure cooker mode to "Pressure."

6. Cook for 30 minutes or until it is cooked.

7. Remove the "snail" from the pressure cooker and rest briefly. Cut it into pieces and serve.

Nutrition: calories 80, fat 5.5, fiber 0, carbs 4.37, protein 4

Puff Rolls

Prep time: 10 minutes

Cooking time: 25 minutes

Servings: 6

Ingredients:

- 7 ounces puff pastry
- 1 teaspoon olive oil
- 1 cup ground beef
- 1 yellow onion
- 1 teaspoon cilantro
- 1 tablespoon cumin
- 1 egg yolk
- 2 tablespoons water
- 1 teaspoon oregano
- ½ teaspoon turmeric
- ½ teaspoon ginger
- 1 teaspoon salt
- ½ tablespoon lemon juice

Directions:

1. Peel the onion and dice it. Combine the diced onion with the cilantro, oregano, turmeric, ginger, and salt.

2. Stir the mixture well and add ground beef. Mix it up.

3. Roll the puff pastry using a rolling pin.

4. Separate it into the medium logs.

5. Add the onion mixture in the puff pastry logs and make long rolls. Whisk the egg yolk with water until blended and add cumin.

6. Sprinkle the pressure cooker with the olive oil inside and transfer the Turkey rolls in the pressure cooker.

7. Brush the logs with the egg mixture.

8. Close the lid, and set the pressure cooker mode to "Pressure," and cook for 25 minutes or until it is done.

9. Remove it from the pressure cooker and rest briefly and serve.

Nutrition: calories 268, fat 18.2, fiber 1, carbs 17.58, protein 9

Garlic Spaghetti

Prep time: 10 minutes

Cooking time: 16 minutes

Servings: 7

Ingredients:

- 6 garlic cloves
- 1 tablespoon garlic powder
- 1 teaspoon onion powder
- 1 tablespoon heavy cream
- 3 tablespoons butter
- 6 ounces Parmesan cheese
- 2 cups chicken stock
- 9 ounces black beans noodles
- ½ cup fresh parsley
- 1 teaspoon white wine
- ½ lemon
- 4 ounces tomatoes
- 1 cup ground chicken

Directions:

1. Cook the black beans noodles to al dente according to the directions on the package. Slice the garlic cloves and combine it with the ground chicken.

2. Add onion powder, garlic powder, cream, white wine, and chicken stock. Blend the mixture.

3. Transfer the mixture to the pressure cooker and sauté it for 6 minutes or until the mixture is cooked.

4. Add the black beans noodles.

5. Chop the tomatoes and add them in the pressure cooker.

6. Grate the Parmesan cheese. Blend the pressure cooker mixture well to not damage the noodles and close the lid.

7. Cook the dish on the pressure mode for 10 minutes. Transfer the cooked dish into the serving plates.

8. Sprinkle it with the grated cheese and serve hot.

Nutrition: calories 302, fat 14, fiber 8.5, carbs 15.5, protein 30.9

Salmon Pie

Prep time: 15 minutes

Cooking time: 35 minutes

Servings: 6

Ingredients:

- 1 pound salmon fillet, boiled
- 1 teaspoon salt
- 7 ounces butter
- 1 cup almond flour
- ½ cup dill
- 1 teaspoon paprika
- 2 tablespoons lemon juice
- 1 teaspoon cilantro
- 5 ounces dried tomatoes
- ¼ cup garlic
- 2 sweet bell peppers
- 1 tablespoon olive oil

Directions:

1. Shred the boiled salmon fillet and sprinkle it with the salt and lemon juice and stir the mixture. Combine the butter with the flour, paprika, and cilantro.

2. Knead the dough. Chop the dill and slice the garlic.

3. Chop the tomatoes and bell peppers. Combine the vegetables together and add the mixture in the shredded salmon.

4. Roll the soft dough using a rolling pin.

5. Spray the pressure cooker with the olive oil inside and transfer the rolled dough there.

6. Add the salmon mixture and flatten it well. Wrap the edges of the dough and close the lid.

7. Cook the pie for 35 minutes on the "Pressure" mode. When the pie is done, let it cool briefly.

8. Remove it from the pressure cooker and slice it. Serve it warm.

Nutrition: calories 515, fat 44.3, fiber 3.6, carbs 11.7, protein 16.8

Onion French Soup

Prep time: 15 minutes

Cooking time: 25 minutes

Servings: 6

Ingredients:

- 1 pound yellow onions
- 1 cup cream
- 4 cups beef stock
- 1 teaspoon salt
- 1 teaspoon ground black pepper
- 1 teaspoon turmeric
- ½ teaspoon nutmeg
- 1 teaspoon cilantro
- ½ teaspoon white pepper
- 1 medium carrot
- 2 ounces unsalted butter

Directions:

1. Peel the onions and carrot. Dice the onion and grate the carrot.

2. Combine the vegetables together and sprinkle the mixture with the salt, ground black pepper, turmeric, nutmeg, cilantro, and white pepper.

3. Blend the mixture.

4. Add the unsalted butter in the pressure cooker and melt it. Add the onion mixture and sauté the vegetables until they are golden brown, stirring frequently.

5. Add beef stock and cream. Stir the mixture well and set the pressure cooker mode to "Sauté." Close the lid and cook the soup for 15 minutes.

6. When the cooking time ends, remove the soup from the pressure cooker and let it cool briefly.

7. Ladle it into the serving bowls and serve it.

Nutrition: calories 277, fat 23.8, fiber 2, carbs 11.58, protein 5

Gnocchi

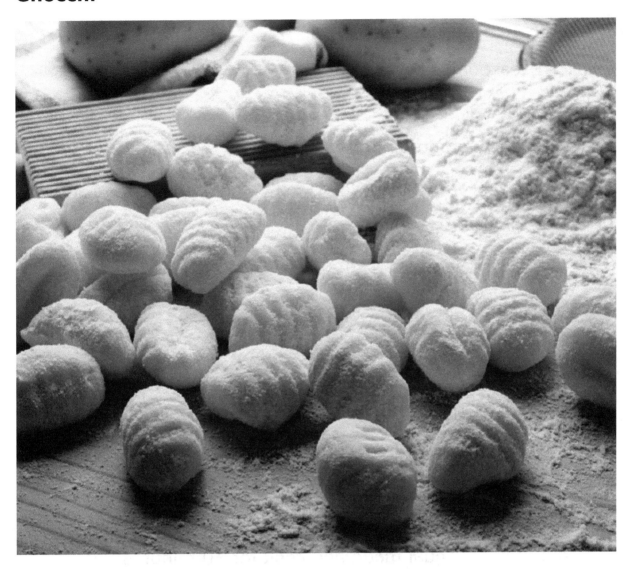

Prep time: 10 minutes

Cooking time: 15 minutes

Servings: 4

Ingredients:

- 8 ounces turnip, flaked

- ½ cup coconut flour

- 1 teaspoon salt

- 4 cups of water

- 1 teaspoon oregano

- ½ teaspoon white pepper

- 1 teaspoon paprika

Directions:

1. Transfer the turnip in the pressure cooker.

2. Add coconut flour, 1 cup of water, salt, oregano, paprika, and white pepper.

3. Stir the mixture gently and close the lid.

4. Set the manual mode and cook for 10 minutes.

5. Blend well and remove it from the pressure cooker.

6. Knead the dough and separate it into the small balls, or gnocchi. Pour 3 cups of the water in the pressure cooker and preheat it.

7. Transfer the gnocchi to the preheated water and stir the mixture well. Close the lid, and set the pressure cooker mode to "Steam."

8. Cook for 7 to 10 minutes or until they are cooked.

9. Remove the dish from the pressure cooker and transfer to the serving plate. Chill it briefly and add your favorite sauce.

Nutrition: calories 89, fat 2.7, fiber 7.5, carbs 13.4, protein 3.7

Mozzarella Pie

Prep time: 15 minutes

Cooking time: 30 minutes

Servings: 8

Ingredients:

- 1 pound rutabaga
- 8 ounces sliced bacon
- 1 onion
- ½ cup cream
- 1 tablespoon olive oil
- 1 teaspoon salt
- 1 teaspoon cilantro
- 1 teaspoon oregano
- ½ teaspoon red chili pepper
- 5 ounces Mozzarella cheese

Directions:

1. Slice the bacon and sprinkle it with the salt and cilantro and stir the mixture.

2. Peel the rutabaga and slice it. Spray the pressure cooker with the olive oil inside. Add half of the sliced bacon into the pressure cooker.

3. Add the sliced rutabaga and sprinkle it with the oregano and red chili pepper. Peel the onion and slice it. Slice the Mozzarella cheese.

4. Add the sliced ingredients in the pressure cooker pie. Pour the cream.

5. Cover the pie with the second half of the sliced bacon and close the lid. Set the pressure cooker mode to "Pressure," and cook for 30 minutes.

6. Release the pressure and check if the pie is cooked.

7. Remove the pie from the pressure cooker and chill it well. Cut the cooked dish into pieces and serve.

Nutrition: calories 255, fat 17.7, fiber 1.8, carbs 7.6, protein 16.5

Herbed Chicken Wings

Prep time: 15 minutes

Cooking time: 10 minutes

Servings: 6

Ingredients:

- 12 chicken wings, bones removed
- 1 tablespoon oregano
- 1 teaspoon paprika
- 1 teaspoon turmeric
- ½ teaspoon salt
- 2 tablespoons butter, melted
- 1 teaspoon cayenne pepper
- ½ teaspoon olive oil
- ½ teaspoon minced garlic

Directions:

1. Make the chicken marinade: mix up together oregano, paprika, turmeric, salt, melted butter, cayenne pepper, olive oil, and minced garlic.

2. Whisk the mixture well. Then brush every chicken wing with marinade and leave for 10 minutes to marinate.

3. After this, transfer the chicken wings into the cooker basket and lower the crisp lid.

4. Cook the chicken wings for 10 minutes or until they are light brown.

Nutrition: calories 361, fat 25.8, fiber 0.9, carbs 11.9, protein 19.7

Halloumi Salad with Beef Tenderloins

Prep time: 15 minutes

Cooking time: 10 minutes

Servings: 6

Ingredients:

- 7 ounces halloumi cheese
- 1 tablespoon orange juice
- 1 teaspoon sesame oil
- ½ teaspoon cumin
- ½ cup arugula
- 1 pound beef tenderloins
- 1 tablespoon lemon juice
- 1 teaspoon apple cider vinegar
- 1 teaspoon salt
- 1 teaspoon ground white pepper
- 1 tablespoon olive oil
- 1 teaspoon rosemary
- 1 cup romaine lettuce

Directions:

1. Tenderize the beef tenderloins well and cover them with the cumin, lemon juice, apple cider vinegar, ground white pepper, salt, and rosemary.

2. Marinate the meat for at least 10 minutes.

3. Transfer the meat to the pressure cooker and sauté for 10 minutes or until it is cooked. Flip it into another side from time to time.

4. Chop the beef tenderloins roughly and transfer them to the serving bowl. Tear the lettuce and add it to the meat bowl.

5. Slice the halloumi cheese and sprinkle it with the sesame oil.

6. Chop the arugula. Add the ingredients to the meat mixture.

7. Sprinkle the salad with the orange juice and mix well. Serve the salad immediately.

Nutrition: calories 289, fat 16.9, fiber 0, carbs 4.53, protein 29

Basil Pho

Prep time: 15 minutes

Cooking time: 32 minutes

Servings: 9

Ingredients:

- 5 cups of water
- 4 ounces scallions
- 3 ounces shallot
- 1 teaspoon salt
- 1 teaspoon paprika
- ½ tablespoon red chili flakes
- 1 teaspoon ground white pepper
- ⅓ cup fresh basil
- 1 tablespoon garlic sauce
- 2 medium onions
- ½ lime
- 1 teaspoon nutmeg
- 2 pounds of chicken breast

Directions:

1. Peel the onions and slice them. Place the sliced onions in the pressure cooker.

2. Chop the shallot and scallions and add them in the pressure cooker too.

3. Sprinkle the mixture with the ground white pepper, chili flakes, paprika, salt, and nutmeg. Stir the mixture and sauté it for 30 seconds.

4. Add water and the chicken breast. Close the lid and cook the mixture at the pressure mode for 30 minutes.

5. When the cooking time ends, release the remaining pressure and remove the chicken from the water.

6. Strain the water using a colander. Shred the chicken.

7. Add the shredded chicken in the serving bowls.

8. Sprinkle the dish with the garlic sauce. Squeeze lime juice from the lime and add the liquid to the dish. Stir it gently and serve immediately.

Nutrition: calories 139, fat 2.7, fiber 1.2, carbs 5.6, protein 22.2

Butter Asparagus Pie

Prep time: 15 minutes

Cooking time: 30 minutes

Servings: 8

Ingredients:

- 10 ounces butter
- 3 cups almond flour
- 1 egg
- 1 teaspoon salt
- 1 pound asparagus
- 2 tablespoons olive oil
- ½ cup pork rind
- 1 teaspoon paprika
- ½ cup dill

Directions:

1. Combine the soft butter, almond flour, and egg together in a mixing bowl. Knead the dough until smooth.

2. Chop the asparagus and dill. Combine the chopped vegetables together.

3. Sprinkle the mixture with the salt, half of the pork rinds, and paprika. Blend the mixture. Transfer the dough to the pressure cooker and flatten it well.

4. Add the chopped asparagus mixture. Sprinkle the pie with the pork rinds.

5. Sprinkle the pie with the olive oil and close the lid. Cook the pie at the pressure mode for 30 minutes.

6. When the dish is cooked, release the remaining pressure and let the pie rest. Cut it into pieces and serve.

Nutrition: calories 622, fat 58, fiber 6.2, carbs 11.6, protein 7.4

Enoki Mushroom Soup

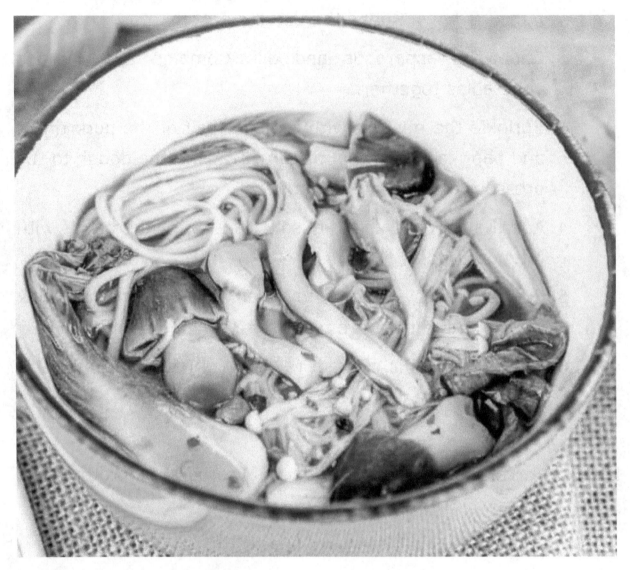

Prep time: 15 minutes

Cooking time: 50 minutes

Servings: 8

Ingredients:

- 1 cup Enoki mushrooms

- 7 cups of water

- 1 cup dill

- 4 tablespoons salsa

- 1 jalapeno pepper

- ⅓ cup cream

- 2 teaspoons salt

- 1 teaspoon white pepper

- 1 white onion

- 1 sweet red bell pepper

- 1 pound chicken breast

- 1 teaspoon soy sauce

Directions:

1. Place Enoki mushrooms in the pressure cooker.

2. Chop the chicken breast and add it in the pressure cooker. Add water and cook the mushrooms at the pressure mode for 35 minutes.

3. Meanwhile, chop the dill and jalapeno peppers. Slice the onions and chop the bell pepper.

4. Add the vegetables to bean mixture and close the lid. Set the pressure cooker mode to "Pressure," and cook for 15 minutes.

5. Sprinkle the soup with the cream, salsa, white pepper, and soy sauce.

6. Stir the soup and cook it for 5 minutes.

7. Remove the soup from the pressure cooker and let it rest briefly. Ladle the soup into the serving bowls.

Nutrition: calories 101, fat 2.3, fiber 1.6, carbs 6.7, protein 13.9

Mushroom Cream Soup

Prep time: 20 minutes

Cooking time: 40 minutes

Servings: 6

Ingredients:

- 1 cup cream
- 6 cups of water
- ¼ cup garlic
- 1 teaspoon salt
- 9 ounces cremini mushrooms
- 1 teaspoon butter
- 5 ounces shallot
- 3 ounces rutabaga
- 2 ounces celery
- 1 teaspoon fresh thyme leaves

Directions:

1. Peel the garlic and slice it. Slice the cremini mushrooms and combine them with the sliced garlic.

2. Toss the mixture into the pressure cooker and sprinkle it with the butter.

3. Sauté the mixture for 7 minutes, stirring frequently. Peel the rutabaga and chop them. Add the chopped rutabaga into the mushroom mixture.

4. Chop the celery and shallot. Add the chopped ingredients into the pressure cooker. Sprinkle the mixture with salt, cream, and water.

5. Chop the fresh thyme leaves and stir the mixture. Close the lid, and set the pressure cooker mode to "Pressure." Cook for 30 minutes.

6. When the cooking time ends, unplug the pressure cooker and blend the soup using a hand mixer.

7. When you get a creamy texture, remove a blender from the soup. Ladle it into the bowls.

Nutrition: calories 75, fat 3, fiber 0.9, carbs 10.4, protein 2.6

Cauliflower Cottage Slice

Prep time: 15 minutes

Cooking time: 25 minutes

Servings: 8

Ingredients:

- 1 pound cauliflower florets
- 1 tablespoon salt
- 7 ounces filo pastry sheets
- 2 tablespoons butter
- 7 eggs
- 8 ounces Parmesan cheese
- ⅓ cup cottage cheese
- 1 tablespoon paprika
- ½ teaspoon nutmeg
- 1 tablespoon olive oil
- ¼ cup cream

Directions:

1. Wash the cauliflower, and chop the florets and sprinkle them with salt. Add the eggs in a mixing bowl and whisk them.

2. Add cottage cheese and paprika and stir the mixture. Add nutmeg and cream.

3. Combine all the ingredients together in a mixing bowl and mix well. Spray the filo pastry sheets with the olive oil and transfer them into the pressure cooker.

4. Add the cauliflower filling and close the lid.

5. Cook the dish on the "Pressure" mode for 25 minutes.

6. When the slice is cooked, release the remaining pressure and let the dish rest briefly. Slice and serve.

Nutrition: calories 407, fat 27.5, fiber 2, carbs 21.13, protein 19

Turkey Apple Salad

Prep time: 15 minutes

Cooking time: 30 minutes

Servings: 8

Ingredients:

- 8 ounces turkey breast
- 1 cup arugula
- ½ cup lettuce
- 2 tablespoons orange juice
- 1 teaspoon sesame oil
- 1 tablespoon sesame seeds
- 1 tablespoon apple cider vinegar
- 1 teaspoon butter
- ½ teaspoon ground black pepper
- 7 ounces red apples
- ¼ cup walnuts
- ½ lime
- 2 cucumbers

- 1 tablespoon mustard

- 1 teaspoon liquid honey

Directions:

1. Sprinkle the turkey breast with the apple cider vinegar, ground black pepper, and mustard. Blend the mixture.

2. Transfer the meat to the pressure cooker.

3. Add butter and cook it on the "Pressure" mode for 25 minutes. Remove the meat from the pressure cooker and let it chill well.

4. Meanwhile, sprinkle the apples with the liquid honey and walnuts.

5. Transfer the apples to the pressure cooker and cook the fruits for 5 minutes at the pressure mode.

6. Remove the apples and chill them.

7. Tear the lettuce and arugula and place them in the mixing bowl. Add sesame oil and chop the cucumbers.

8. Add the chopped cucumbers in the mixture. Squeeze the lime juice onto the salad. Chop the cooked apples and chicken and place them in the salad mixture.

9. Add orange juice and sesame seeds. Stir the salad carefully using a wooden spoon. Serve immediately.

Nutrition: calories 198, fat 16.1, fiber 1, carbs 6.97, protein 7

Ground Meat Chop

Prep time: 15 minutes

Cooking time: 20 minutes

Servings: 4

Ingredients:

- 1 cup cauliflower rice
- 2 cups ground beef
- ¼ cup tomato paste
- 1 tablespoon ground black pepper
- 3 cups of water
- 1 tablespoon olive oil
- 1 tablespoon lemon juice
- 1 tablespoon cilantro
- 1 teaspoon salt
- ¼ cup of soy sauce
- 1 teaspoon sliced garlic

Directions:

1. Place the ground beef in the pressure cooker.

2. Add the ground black pepper, cilantro, salt, and sliced garlic.

3. Sprinkle the mixture with olive oil and stir. Set the pressure cooker mode to "Sauté" the meat for 6 minutes.

4. Stir the ground meat mixture well. Add cauliflower rice and combine.

5. Add tomato paste, water, and lemon juice. Stir the mixture and close the lid. Set the pressure cooker mode to "Saute" and cook for 20 minutes.

6. When the dish is cooked, sprinkle it with the soy sauce and stir. Transfer the dish to serving bowls.

Nutrition: calories 194, fat 11.9, fiber 1.9, carbs 7, protein 15.5

Provolone Pepper Soup

Prep time: 10 minutes

Cooking time: 18 minutes

Servings: 4

Ingredients:

- 3 oz bacon, chopped
- 10 oz chicken fillet, chopped
- 3 oz Provolone cheese, grated
- 1 tablespoon cream cheese
- 1 white onion, diced
- ½ teaspoon salt
- ½ teaspoon ground black pepper
- 1 teaspoon dried parsley
- 1 garlic clove, diced
- 4 cups of water

Directions:

1. Place the chopped bacon in the instant pot and cook it for 5 minutes on sauté mode.

2. Stir it from time to time to avoid burning.

3.   After this, transfer the cooked bacon in the plate and dry little with the paper towel.

4.   Then add onion and diced garlic in the instant pot.

5.   Sauté the vegetables for 2 minutes and add chicken and cream cheese. Stir well and sauté the ingredients for 5 minutes.

6.   After this, add salt, ground black pepper, dried parsley, water, and Provolone cheese. Stir the soup mixture well.

7.   Close the lid and cook the soup for 5 minutes on manual mode (high pressure). Then make a quick pressure release. Add the cooked bacon in the soup.

8.   Stir the cooked soup well before serving.

Nutrition value/serving: calories 346, fat 20.7, fiber 0.7, carbs 3.8, protein 34.4

Jalapeno Garlic Soup

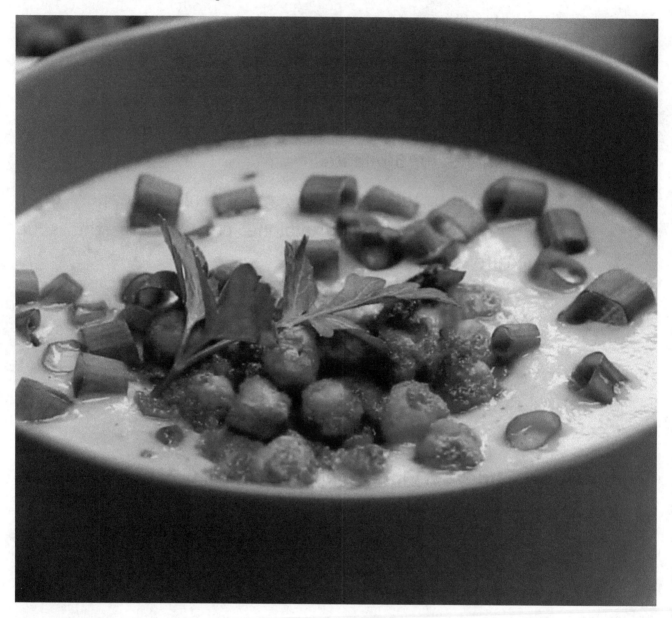

Prep time: 10 minutes

Cooking time: 20 minutes

Servings: 4

Ingredients:

- ½ cup ground pork

- 1 teaspoon garlic powder

- 1 bell pepper, diced

- 1 jalapeno pepper, sliced

- 1 teaspoon coconut oil

- 1 tomato, chopped

- ½ teaspoon salt

- 1 teaspoon thyme

- 4 cups of water

Directions:

1. Put the coconut oil in the instant pot and preheat it on Saute mode.

2. When the coconut oil starts shimmering, add bell pepper and jalapeno pepper.

3. Cook the vegetables for 1 minute and stir them.

4. Add ground pork, garlic powder, tomato, salt, and thyme.

5. Stir well and sauté the ingredients for 2 minutes.

6. Then add water and close the lid.

7. Cook the jalapeno soup for 5 minutes on Manual mode (high pressure).

8. Then allow the natural pressure release for 5 minutes.

Nutrition value/serving: calories 142, fat 9.4, fiber 0.9, carbs 3.7, protein 10.7

Eggplant Lasagna with Mozzarella

Prep time: 15 minutes

Cooking time: 10 minutes

Servings: 6

Ingredients:

- 2 eggplants, peeled, sliced
- 1 cup ground pork
- 3 tablespoons marinara sauce
- 1 white onion, diced
- 1 oz fresh basil, chopped
- ½ cup Ricotta cheese
- ½ cup Mozzarella, shredded
- ½ teaspoon dried oregano
- ¼ teaspoon salt
- 1 cup water, for cooking

Directions:

1. In the mixing bowl combine together ground pork, diced onion, basil, and dried oregano.

2. Add salt and stir the meat mixture well with the help of the spoon.

3.   Line the baking pan with paper foil.

4.   Then place the sliced eggplants in the baking pan to make the layer.

5.   Sprinkle the eggplants with marinara sauce.

6.   Top the marinara sauce with ground pork mixture.

7.   Then spread the mixture with Ricotta cheese and shredded Mozzarella.

8.   Cover the lasagna with foil.

9.   Pour water in the instant pot and insert the trivet.

10.   Place the lasagna on the trivet and close the lid.

11.   Cook the lasagna for 10 minutes on manual mode (high pressure).

12.   Then make a quick pressure release.

13.   Cool the cooked lasagna little before serving.

Nutrition value/serving: calories 251, fat 13.5, fiber 7.2, carbs 14.9, protein 18.7

Keto Cauliflower Soup

Prep time: 15 minutes

Cooking time: 4 minutes

Servings: 2

Ingredients:

- 1 cup cauliflower, chopped
- 1 oz bacon, chopped, cooked
- 2 oz Cheddar cheese, shredded
- 2 tablespoons cream cheese
- 1 oz leek, chopped
- 1 cup of water
- ½ teaspoon salt
- ½ teaspoon cayenne pepper

Directions:

1. Pour water in the instant pot.

2. Add cauliflower, cream cheese, leek, salt, and cayenne pepper.

3. Close the lid and cook soup mixture for 4 minutes on Manual mode (high pressure).

4. Allow the natural pressure release for 10 minutes.

5.   Then add cheese and stir the soup until it is melted.

6.   With the help of the immersion blender, blend the soup until you get the creamy texture.

7.   Then ladle the soup in the serving bowls and top with bacon.

Nutrition value/serving: calories 248, fat 19, fiber 1.6, carbs 5.7, protein 14.3

Chili Egg Soup

Prep time: 5 minutes

Cooking time: 15 minutes

Servings: 2

Ingredients:

- 2 eggs, beaten
- 2 cups chicken broth
- 1 tablespoon chives, chopped
- ½ teaspoon salt
- ½ teaspoon chili flakes

Directions:

1. Pour chicken broth in the instant pot.
2. Add chives, salt, and chili flakes.
3. Saute the liquid for 10 minutes.
4. Then add beaten eggs and stir the soup well.
5. Cook the soup for 5 minutes more.

Nutrition value/serving: calories 102, fat 5.8, fiber 0.1, carbs 1.3, protein 10.5

Beef Soup

Prep time: 10 minutes

Cooking time: 15 minutes

Servings: 6

Ingredients:

- 1 cup white cabbage, shredded
- ½ cup kale, chopped
- 11 oz beef sirloin, chopped
- ½ teaspoon salt
- 1 teaspoon dried basil
- ½ teaspoon fennel seeds
- ½ teaspoon ground black pepper
- 1 garlic clove, diced
- 1 teaspoon almond butter
- 5 cups of water

Directions:

1. Put almond butter in the instant pot and melt it on sauté mode.

2. Add white cabbage and diced garlic. Cook the vegetables for 5 minutes. Stir them occasionally.

3.   Then add chopped beef sirloin, fennel seeds, ground black pepper, salt, and stir well.

4.   Add basil and water.

5.   Then add kale and close the lid.

6.   Cook the soup on Manual mode (high pressure) for 5 minutes.

7.   Then make a quick pressure release.

Nutrition value/serving: calories 120, fat 4.8, fiber 0.8, carbs 2.1, protein 16.7

Hot Spinach Chowder

Prep time: 10 minutes

Cooking time: 20 minutes

Servings: 4

Ingredients:

- 1 cup fresh spinach, chopped
- ½ cup heavy cream
- 4 oz bacon, chopped, cooked
- 1 teaspoon dried dill
- ½ teaspoon salt
- 4 chicken thighs, skinless, boneless, chopped
- ½ teaspoon cayenne pepper
- ½ teaspoon ground thyme
- 1 teaspoon coconut oil
- 1 teaspoon minced garlic
- 4 cups of water
- ½ cup mushrooms, chopped

Directions:

1. Put coconut oil in the instant pot and melt it on sauté mode.

2. Then add chopped chicken thighs, salt, dill, cayenne pepper, and ground thyme.

3. Stir the chicken well and sauté for 5 minutes.

4. After this, add minced garlic and chopped mushrooms. Stir well and cook for 5 minutes more.

5. Then add heavy cream and water.

6. Then add chopped spinach and bacon. Close the lid and cook the chowder on Manual mode (high pressure) for 10 minutes.

7. Then make a quick pressure release and open the lid.

8. Cool the chowder for 10-15 minutes before serving.

Nutrition value/serving: calories 249, fat 19.4, fiber 0.4, carbs 2, protein 16.4

Butternut Ginger Soup

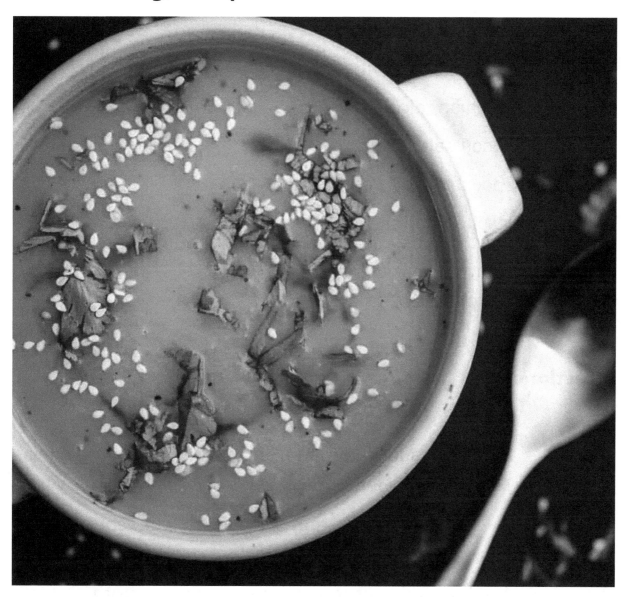

Prep time: 10 minutes

Cooking time: 25 minutes

Servings: 6

Ingredients:

- 2 cups butternut squash, chopped

- 2 garlic cloves, peeled, diced

- 1 teaspoon curry powder

- ½ teaspoon ginger, minced

- 1 white onion, diced

- 1 teaspoon salt

- 1 teaspoon ground paprika

- 1 tablespoon butter

- 5 cups chicken broth

- 2 tablespoons Ricotta cheese

Directions:

1.   Melt butter in sauté mode.

2.   Then add garlic and onion. Saute the vegetables until they are golden brown.

3.   Then add butternut squash, ginger, salt, ground paprika, and ricotta cheese.

4.   Then add curry powder and chicken broth.

5.   Close the lid and cook the soup on manual mode (high pressure) for 15 minutes.

6.   Then make a quick pressure release.

7.   Blend the soup with the help of the immersion blender.

Nutrition value/serving: calories 87, fat 3.6, fiber 1.4, carbs 8.7, protein 5.5

Tortilla Soup

Prep time: 10 minutes

Cooking time: 30 minutes

Servings: 2

Ingredients:

- ½ Poblano pepper, chopped
- ¼ teaspoon minced garlic
- ¼ teaspoon ground coriander
- ½ cup tomatoes, canned
- 1 tablespoon dried cilantro
- ¼ teaspoon salt
- 2 cups chicken broth
- 8 oz chicken breast, skinless, boneless
- 1 tablespoon lemon juice
- 1 teaspoon butter
- ¼ cup Cheddar cheese, shredded
- 2 low carb tortillas, chopped

Directions:

1. Melt butter in sauté mode.

2. When the butter is melted, add chopped Poblano pepper, minced garlic, ground coriander, and dried cilantro.

3. Add chicken breast and cook the ingredients for 10 minutes. Stir them from time to time.

4. After this, add canned tomatoes, salt, and chicken broth.

5. Close the lid and cook the soup on manual mode (high pressure) for 15 minutes.

6. Then make a quick pressure release and open the lid.

7. Add lemon juice and sauté the soup for 5 minutes more.

8. Ladle the soup into the bowls and top with Cheddar cheese and chopped low carb tortillas.

Nutrition value/serving: calories 336, fat 13, fiber 8.3, carbs 16.1, protein 36.2

Steak Zucchini Soup

Prep time: 10 minutes

Cooking time: 25 minutes

Servings: 4

Ingredients:

- ½ teaspoon minced ginger
- ¼ teaspoon minced garlic
- 1 teaspoon coconut oil
- 10 oz beef sirloin steak, chopped
- ½ cup cremini mushrooms, sliced
- 4 cups chicken broth
- ½ teaspoon salt
- 1 zucchini, trimmed
- 1 teaspoon chives, chopped

Directions:

1. Heat up instant pot on sauté mode.

2. Toss coconut oil and melt it.

3. Then add minced ginger and minced garlic. Stir well and add chopped steak.

4. Sauté the mixture for 5 minutes.

5. Meanwhile, with the help of the spiralizer make the zucchini noodles.

6. Add mushrooms in the beef mixture. Then sprinkle it with salt.

7. Add chicken broth and cook the soup on Manual mode (high pressure) for 12 minutes.

8. Then make a quick pressure release and open the lid.

9. Add spiralized noodles and stir the soup. Let it rest for 5 minutes.

10. Top the cooked soup with chives.

Nutrition value/serving: calories 191, fat 7, fiber 0.6, carbs 3.2, protein 27.2

Chili Meat

Prep time: 10 minutes

Cooking time: 3 hours 5 minutes

Servings: 2

Ingredients:

- 9 oz pork shoulder, chopped
- ½ cup salsa Verde
- 1 teaspoon sesame oil
- ½ cup chicken broth
- ¼ teaspoon cayenne pepper
- ¼ teaspoon salt

Directions:

1. Pour sesame oil in the instant pot and preheat it on sauté mode for 3 minutes.

2. Meanwhile, mix up together pork shoulder, cayenne pepper, and salt.

3. Add the pork shoulder in the hot oil and sauté the meat for 2 minutes.

4. Then stir it with the help of the spatula and add chicken broth and salsa Verde.

5.   Close the lid.

6.   Cook the meal on manual (low pressure) for 3 hours.

7.   When the time is over, shred the meat.

Nutrition value/serving: calories 418, fat 30.1, fiber 0.3, carbs 2.9, protein 31.7

Garlic Taco Soup

Prep time: 10 minutes

Cooking time: 25 minutes

Servings: 5

Ingredients:

- 2 cups ground beef
- 1 teaspoon onion powder
- 1 teaspoon taco seasonings
- 1 garlic clove, diced
- 1 teaspoon chili flakes
- 1 teaspoon ground cumin
- 1 tablespoon tomato paste
- ½ cup heavy cream
- 5 cups of water
- 1 teaspoon coconut oil
- 1 tablespoon cream cheese
- 1 jalapeno pepper, sliced

Directions:

1. Toss the coconut oil in the instant pot and melt it on sauté mode.

2. Add ground beef and onion powder.

3. After this, add taco seasonings and diced garlic. Mix up the ingredients well.

4. Then sprinkle the meat mixture with chili flakes and ground cumin.

5. Saute the ground beef for 10 minutes. Mix it up with the help of the spatula every 3 minutes.

6. Then add tomato paste, heavy cream, and water.

7. Add sliced jalapeno pepper and close the lid.

8. Cook the soup on Manual (high pressure) for 10 minutes.

9. Then allow the natural pressure release for 10 minutes and ladle the soup into the bowls.

Nutrition value/serving: calories 170, fat 12.7, fiber 0.3, carbs 2.4, protein 11.2

Chicken Chipotle Soup

Prep time: 10 minutes

Cooking time: 32 minutes

Servings: 4

Ingredients:

- 1-pound chicken fillet
- ½ white onion, chopped
- 1 bell pepper, chopped
- 1 jalapeno pepper, chopped
- 1 tablespoon avocado oil
- 1 tablespoon tomato paste
- 1 teaspoon apple cider vinegar
- 1 teaspoon chipotle pepper
- ½ teaspoon garlic powder
- ½ teaspoon ground cumin
- ½ teaspoon ground coriander
- ½ teaspoon ground paprika
- 1/3 teaspoon salt
- 1 teaspoon dried oregano
- 4 cups of water

Directions:

1. Pour avocado oil in the instant pot.

2. Add white onion, bell pepper, and jalapeno pepper.

3. Saute the vegetables on sauté mode for 5 minutes.

4. Meanwhile, in the shallow bowl combine together garlic powder, cumin, coriander, paprika, salt, and dried oregano.

5. Add the spices in the vegetables.

6. Then add tomato paste, chipotle pepper, and apple cider vinegar.

7. Add water and chicken fillet.

8. Close the lid and cook enchilada soup on Manual mode (high pressure) for 25 minutes.

9. Then make a quick pressure release and open the lid.

10. With the help of 2 forks shred the chicken fillet and stir the soup.

Nutrition value/serving: calories 244, fat 9.1, fiber 1.4, carbs 5.5, protein 33.7

Creamy Cheddar Soup

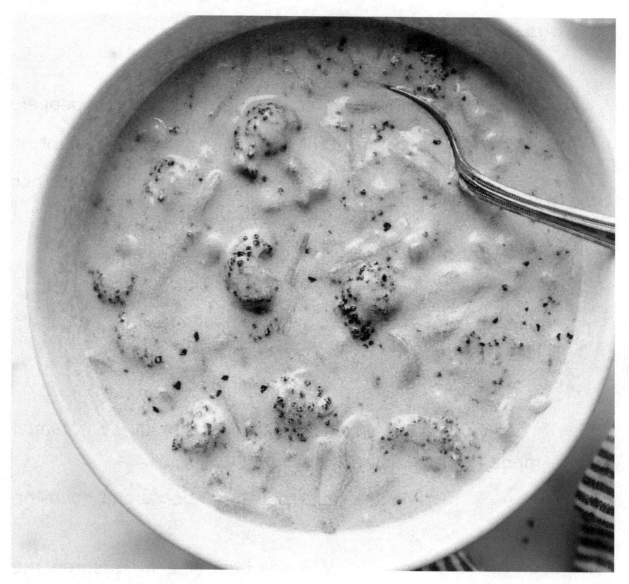

Prep time: 10 minutes

Cooking time: 15 minutes

Servings: 2

Ingredients:

- 1 tablespoon cream cheese

- 1 oz bacon, chopped, cooked

- 2 oz Cheddar cheese, shredded

- 2 cups cauliflower, chopped

- ½ teaspoon salt

- 1 teaspoon dried oregano

- 2 cups chicken broth

- ½ teaspoon ground nutmeg

- ½ medium white onion, diced

Directions:

1. Place onion and cream cheese in the instant pot.

2. Cook the ingredients on sauté mode until onion is light brown.

3. Then add chopped cauliflower, salt, dried oregano, and ground nutmeg.

4. Cook the vegetables for 3 minutes.

5. Then stir them well and add chicken broth.

6. Cook the soup on Manual (High pressure) for 4 minutes.

7. Then make a quick pressure release and open the lid.

8. With the help of immersion blender, blend the soup until smooth.

9.   Ladle the soup in the bowls and top with Cheddar cheese and cook bacon.

Nutrition value/serving: calories 286, fat 18.8, fiber 3.2, carbs 9.7, protein 19.9

Sausage Soup

Prep time: 10 minutes

Cooking time: 17 minutes

Servings: 4

Ingredients:

- 3 cups of water
- 9 oz sausages, chopped
- 2 oz Parmesan
- ½ cup heavy cream
- 2 cups kale, chopped
- ½ teaspoon ground black pepper
- ¼ onion, diced
- 1 teaspoon dried basil
- 1 tablespoon olive oil

Directions:

1. Pour olive oil in the instant pot and add the onion.

2. Saute the onion for 3 minutes.

3. Then stir well and add sausages. Mix up well and cook them for 3 minutes.

4. After this, add water, kale, basil, and ground black pepper.

5. Saute the mixture for 8 minutes.

6. Then add heavy cream and Parmesan.

7. Close the lid and cook the soup on manual mode (high pressure) for 3 minutes. Then make a quick pressure release.

8. Let the cooked kale soup cool for 10-15 minutes before serving.

Nutrition value/serving: calories 364, fat 30.2, fiber 0.7, carbs 5.3, protein 18.4

Bone Broth Soup

Prep time: 7 minutes

Cooking time: 10 minutes

Servings: 2

Ingredients:

- 1 eggplant, trimmed, chopped
- 2 cups bone broth
- ¼ cup carrot, grated
- 1 tablespoon butter
- ½ teaspoon salt
- 1 teaspoon dried dill

Directions:

1. In the mixing bowl combine together eggplants and salt. Leave the vegetables for 5 minutes.

2. Meanwhile, toss the butter in the instant pot and melt it on sauté mode.

3. Add grated carrot and cook it for 2 minutes.

4. Meanwhile, dry the eggplants.

5. Add them in the carrot and stir. Sprinkle the vegetables with dried dill.

6.   Then add bone broth and close the lid.

7.   Cook the soup for 5 minutes on Manual mode (high pressure). Then make a quick pressure release.

Nutrition value/serving: calories 200, fat 6.2, fiber 8.5, carbs 15.1, protein 22.5

Celery Chicken Soup

Prep time: 10 minutes

Cooking time: 15 minutes

Servings: 5

Ingredients:

- 1 white onion, diced
- ½ cup celery stalk, chopped
- ½ teaspoon minced garlic
- 1 teaspoon olive oil
- 1-pound chicken breast, cooked, shredded
- 4 cups chicken broth
- 1 tablespoon buffalo sauce

Directions:

1. In the instant pot bowl mix up together onion, minced garlic, and olive oil.

2. Cook the ingredients on sauté mode for 4 minutes.

3. Then stir them well and add shredded chicken breast.

4. Add chicken broth and buffalo sauce. Mix up well.

5. Cook the soup on soup mode for 10 minutes.

Nutrition value/serving: calories 154, fat 4.3, fiber 0.7, carbs 3.4, protein 23.4

Cream & Vegetable Stew

Prep time: 10 minutes

Cooking time: 25 minutes

Servings: 2

Ingredients:

- 4 oz sausages, chopped
- ½ cup savoy cabbage, chopped
- 2 oz turnip, chopped
- ¼ cup bok choy, chopped
- 1 teaspoon ground cumin
- ¼ teaspoon fennel seeds
- ½ cup heavy cream
- ½ teaspoon salt
- 1 teaspoon butter

Directions:

1. Preheat the instant pot on sauté mode for 2 minutes.

2. Toss the butter inside and melt it.

3. After this, add sausages and cook them for 5 minutes on sauté mode. Stir them from time to time.

4. Then add salt, fennel seeds, ground cumin, and heavy cream.

5. Add savoy cabbage, turnip, and bok choy. Stir the stew well.

6. Cook the stew on stew mode for 15 minutes.

Nutrition value/serving: calories 331, fat 29.4, fiber 1.3, carbs 4.5, protein 12.5

Broccoli Lunch Bowl

Prep time: 10 minutes

Cooking time: 25 minutes

Servings: 2

Ingredients:

- ½ cup broccoli, chopped
- 8 oz chicken fillet, chopped
- 1 green bell pepper, chopped
- 1 teaspoon ground black pepper
- ½ teaspoon dried cilantro
- 1 cup chicken broth
- ½ teaspoon salt
- ½ teaspoon almond butter

Directions:

1. Place almond butter, bell pepper, and broccoli in the instant pot.

2. Cook the ingredients on sauté mode for 5 minutes. Stir them with the help of the spatula from time to time.

3. After this, add chopped chicken fillet, ground black pepper, salt, and cilantro.

4.　Add chicken broth and mix up the meal well.

5.　Close the lid and cook it on stew mode for 20 minutes.

6.　When the meal is cooked, let it rest for 10 minutes before serving.

Nutrition value/serving: calories 289, fat 11.6, fiber 2.1, carbs 7.9, protein 37.4

Cabbage Salad

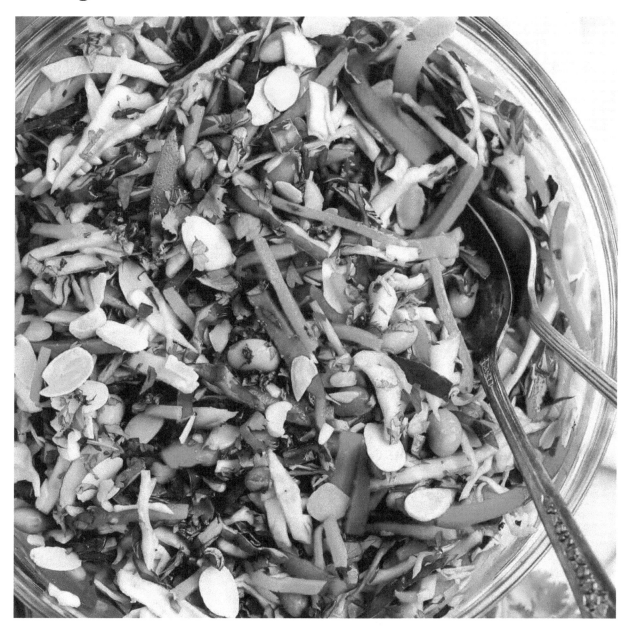

Prep time: 10 minutes

Cooking time: 21 minutes

Servings: 4

Ingredients:

- 1-pound chicken breast, skinless, boneless

- 1 avocado, pitted, peeled

- 4 eggs

- 1 cup lettuce, chopped

- 1 tablespoon lemon juice

- ¼ teaspoon salt

- ½ teaspoon white pepper

- ½ cup white cabbage, shredded

- 4 oz Feta cheese, crumbled

- 1 tablespoon coconut oil

- ½ teaspoon chili flakes

- 1 tablespoon heavy cream

- 1 tablespoon apple cider vinegar

- ½ teaspoon garlic powder

- 1 cup water, for cooking

Directions:

1. Pour water and insert the trivet in the instant pot.

2. Place the eggs on the trivet and close the lid.

3. Cook them in manual mode (high pressure) for 5 minutes. Then make a quick pressure release.

4. Cool the eggs in ice water. Then peel the eggs.

5. Cut the eggs and avocado into the wedges.

6. After this, rub the chicken breast with lemon juice, salt, and coconut oil.

7. Place the chicken breast in the instant pot and cook it on sauté mode for 7 minutes from each side. The cooked chicken should be light brown.

8. Make the sauce: whisk together chili flakes, olive oil, heavy cream, apple cider vinegar, and garlic powder.

9. In the big salad bowl combine together lettuce, eggs, avocado, white pepper, white cabbage, and crumbled feta.

10. Chop the cooked chicken roughly and add in the salad. Shake the salad well.

11. Then sprinkle the cooked cobb salad with sauce.

Nutrition value/serving: calories 417, fat 27.9, fiber 3.8, carbs 7.4, protein 34.9

Cucumber and Lobster Salad

Prep time: 10 minutes

Cooking time: 4 minutes

Servings: 4

Ingredients:

- 4 lobster tails, peeled
- 1 teaspoon avocado oil
- ¼ teaspoon salt
- 2 cucumbers, chopped
- ¼ cup whipped cream
- 1 tablespoon apple cider vinegar
- 1 teaspoon dried dill
- ½ cup celery stalk, chopped
- 1 cup water, for cooking

Directions:

1. Pour water and insert the trivet in the instant pot.

2. Arrange the lobster tails on the trivet and cook them on Manual mode (high pressure) for 4 minutes. Then make a quick pressure release.

3.   Cool the cooked lobster tails little and chop them roughly.

4.   Place the chopped lobster tails in the salad bowl.

5.   Add cucumbers, dried ill, and celery stalk.

6.   After this, make the salad sauce: in the shallow bowl combine together salt, avocado oil, whipped cream, dill, and apple cider vinegar.

7.   Sprinkle the salad with sauce and mix up it well with the help of 2 spoons.

Nutrition value/serving: calories 139, fat 3.7, fiber 1, carbs 6.3, protein 1.3

Italian Salad

Prep time: 5 minutes

Cooking time: 5 minutes

Servings: 2

Ingredients:

- 8 oz shrimps, peeled
- 1 teaspoon Italian seasonings
- 1 teaspoon olive oil
- ½ cup cherry tomatoes, halved
- ¼ teaspoon chili flakes
- ½ teaspoon coconut oil

Directions:

1. Toss coconut oil in the instant pot.

2. Melt it on sauté mode and add peeled shrimps.

3. Cook the shrimps for 1 minute from each side.

4. Then place the shrimps in the bowl.

5. Add chili flakes, Italian seasonings, halved cherry tomatoes, and olive oil.

6. Shake the salad before serving.

Nutrition value/serving: calories 173, fat 5.5, fiber 0.5, carbs 3.5, protein 26.2

Egg Salad and Cheddar with Dill

Prep time: 15 minutes

Cooking time: 4 minutes

Servings: 3

Ingredients:

- 3 eggs
- 2 tablespoons cream cheese
- 1 tablespoon dried dill
- ½ cup Cheddar cheese, shredded
- ¼ teaspoon minced garlic
- 1 cup water, for cooking

Directions:

1. Pour water and insert rack in the instant pot.

2. Place the eggs in the instant pot, close the lid and cook them for 4 minutes on Manual mode (high pressure). Then make a quick pressure release.

3. Cool the eggs in cold water for 10 minutes.

4. After this, peel the eggs and grate them.

5. In the mixing bowl combine together grated eggs, shredded cheese, minced garlic, dill, and cream cheese.

6. Mix up the salad well.

Nutrition value/serving: calories 165, fat 13, fiber 0.1, carbs 1.4, protein 11

Cream Cheese Salad

Prep time: 10 minutes

Cooking time: 2 minutes

Servings: 2

Ingredients:

- 10 oz crab meat
- 1 tablespoon sour cream
- 1 tablespoon cream
- ¼ teaspoon minced garlic
- 1 tablespoon cream cheese
- ½ teaspoon lime juice
- ½ red onion, diced
- ¼ cup fresh cilantro, chopped
- ¼ cup fresh spinach, chopped
- ¼ teaspoon salt
- ¼ teaspoon ground cumin
- 1 cup water, for cooking

Directions:

1. Pour water in the instant pot.

2. Line the trivet with the paper foil and insert the instant pot.

3. Place the crab meat on the trivet and cook it on Manual mode (high pressure) for 2 minutes. Then make a quick pressure release and remove the crab meat from the instant pot.

4. Chop it and place it in the salad bowl.

5. Add diced onion, spinach, and cilantro.

6. In the shallow bowl make the salad dressing: whisk together sour cream, cream, minced garlic, cream cheese, and lime juice.

7. Then add salt and ground cumin.

8. Add the dressing in the salad and stir it well.

Nutrition value/serving: calories 175, fat 6, fiber 0.8, carbs 6.4, protein 18.9

Chicken Paprika

Prep time: 10 minutes

Cooking time: 25 minutes

Servings: 2

Ingredients:

- 2 chicken thighs, skinless, boneless
- 2 tablespoons ground paprika
- 1 tablespoon almond meal
- 1 teaspoon tomato paste
- ½ teaspoon dried celery root
- ½ cup heavy cream
- 1 tablespoon butter
- ½ teaspoon salt
- ½ teaspoon white pepper
- ¼ teaspoon ground nutmeg
- 1 tablespoon lemon juice

Directions:

1. Melt butter in sauté mode.

2.   Meanwhile, rub the chicken thighs with salt and white pepper.

3.   Cook the chicken thighs on sauté mode for 4 minutes from each side.

4.   Meanwhile, in the mixing bowl combine together almond meal, dried celery root, and ground nutmeg.

5.   In the separated bowl combine together heavy cream, tomato paste, and lemon juice.

6.   Pour the heavy cream liquid in the chicken.

7.   Then add almond meal mixture and stir gently.

8.   Cook the meal on meat mode for 15 minutes.

Nutrition value/serving: calories 476, fat 30.3, fiber 3.3, carbs 6.5, protein 44.8

Conclusion

Being an ideal remedy both for instant pot beginners and seasoned instant pot individuals this instant pot recipe book raises your everyday food preparation. It makes you look like a pro and prepare like a pro. Thanks to the Instant Pot component, this recipe book aids you with preparing easy as well as yummy dishes for any budget plan. Satisfy every person with passionate dinners, nutritious breakfasts, sweetest desserts, as well as fun snacks. Despite if you cook for one or prepare bigger parts-- there's an option for any type of feasible cooking scenario. Improve your methods on just how to cook in one of the most reliable means making use of just your instant pot, this recipe book, and also some patience to discover fast. Useful pointers and techniques are discreetly incorporated into every dish to make your family members request new meals time and time again. Vegetarian alternatives, options for meat-eaters and also highly pleasing suggestions to unify the whole family members at the exact same table. Consuming in the house is a shared experience, as well as it can be so great to meet all together at the end of the day. Master your Instantaneous Pot and also maximize this new experience starting today!

CPSIA information can be obtained
at www.ICGtesting.com
Printed in the USA
BVHW05050020621
608546BV00014B/2391